Instant Pot Tasty Recipes for Family

The best collection of Instant Pot recipes

Ann Westinghouse

Sommario

Introduction

This total as well as helpful guide to instantaneous pot food preparation with over 1000 dishes for morning meal, dinner, supper, and also treats! This is just one of one of the most comprehensive split second pot recipe books ever before released thanks to its range and also precise guidelines. Innovative dishes and also classics, modern take on household's most enjoyed dishes-- all this is delicious, basic as well as naturally as healthy and balanced as it can be. Modification the way you cook with these cutting-edge split second pot guidelines. Required a brand-new supper or a treat? Below you are! Best instant pot dishes collaborated in a few basic actions, even a newbie can do it! The instantaneous pot specifies the way you cook each day. This immediate pot cookbook assists you make the outright most out of your weekly menu.

The only instant pot book you will certainly ever before need with the supreme collection of recipes will assist you towards a less complex and also much healthier kitchen experience. If you wish to save time cooking dishes extra effectively, if you wish to offer your family members food that can please even the pickiest eater, you are in the right area! Master your immediate pot and make your food preparation needs suit your hectic way of living.

Mushroom Cream Soup

Prep time: 20 minutes
Cooking time: 40 minutes
Servings: 6

Ingredients:

- 1 cup cream
- 6 cups of water
- ¼ cup garlic
- 1 teaspoon salt
- 9 ounces cremini mushrooms
- 1 teaspoon butter
- 5 ounces shallot
- 3 ounces rutabaga
- 2 ounces celery
- 1 teaspoon fresh thyme leaves

Directions:

1. Peel the garlic and slice it. Slice the cremini mushrooms and combine them with the sliced garlic.
2. Toss the mixture into the pressure cooker and sprinkle it with the butter.

3. Sauté the mixture for 7 minutes, stirring frequently. Peel the rutabaga and chop them. Add the chopped rutabaga into the mushroom mixture.
4. Chop the celery and shallot. Add the chopped ingredients into the pressure cooker. Sprinkle the mixture with salt, cream, and water.
5. Chop the fresh thyme leaves and stir the mixture. Close the lid, and set the pressure cooker mode to "Pressure." Cook for 30 minutes.
6. When the cooking time ends, unplug the pressure cooker and blend the soup using a hand mixer.
7. When you get a creamy texture, remove a blender from the soup. Ladle it into the bowls.

Nutrition: calories 75, fat 3, fiber 0.9, carbs 10.4, protein 2.6

Cauliflower Cottage Slice

Prep time: 15 minutes
Cooking time: 25 minutes
Servings: 8

Ingredients:

- 1 pound cauliflower florets
- 1 tablespoon salt
- 7 ounces filo pastry sheets
- 2 tablespoons butter
- 7 eggs
- 8 ounces Parmesan cheese
- ⅓ cup cottage cheese
- 1 tablespoon paprika
- ½ teaspoon nutmeg
- 1 tablespoon olive oil
- ¼ cup cream

Directions:

1. Wash the cauliflower, and chop the florets and sprinkle them with salt. Add the eggs in a mixing bowl and whisk them.

2. Add cottage cheese and paprika and stir the mixture. Add nutmeg and cream.
3. Combine all the ingredients together in a mixing bowl and mix well. Spray the filo pastry sheets with the olive oil and transfer them into the pressure cooker.
4. Add the cauliflower filling and close the lid.
5. Cook the dish on the "Pressure" mode for 25 minutes.
6. When the slice is cooked, release the remaining pressure and let the dish rest briefly. Slice and serve.

Nutrition: calories 407, fat 27.5, fiber 2, carbs 21.13, protein 19

Turkey Apple Salad

Prep time: 15 minutes
Cooking time: 30 minutes
Servings: 8

Ingredients:

- 8 ounces turkey breast
- 1 cup arugula
- ½ cup lettuce
- 2 tablespoons orange juice
- 1 teaspoon sesame oil
- 1 tablespoon sesame seeds
- 1 tablespoon apple cider vinegar
- 1 teaspoon butter
- ½ teaspoon ground black pepper
- 7 ounces red apples
- ¼ cup walnuts
- ½ lime
- 2 cucumbers
- 1 tablespoon mustard
- 1 teaspoon liquid honey

Directions:

1. Sprinkle the turkey breast with the apple cider vinegar, ground black pepper, and mustard. Blend the mixture.
2. Transfer the meat to the pressure cooker.
3. Add butter and cook it on the "Pressure" mode for 25 minutes. Remove the meat from the pressure cooker and let it chill well.
4. Meanwhile, sprinkle the apples with the liquid honey and walnuts.
5. Transfer the apples to the pressure cooker and cook the fruits for 5 minutes at the pressure mode.
6. Remove the apples and chill them.
7. Tear the lettuce and arugula and place them in the mixing bowl. Add sesame oil and chop the cucumbers.
8. Add the chopped cucumbers in the mixture. Squeeze the lime juice onto the salad. Chop the cooked apples and chicken and place them in the salad mixture.
9. Add orange juice and sesame seeds. Stir the salad carefully using a wooden spoon. Serve immediately.

Nutrition: calories 198, fat 16.1, fiber 1, carbs 6.97, protein 7

Ground Meat Chop

Prep time: 15 minutes
Cooking time: 20 minutes
Servings: 4

Ingredients:

- 1 cup cauliflower rice
- 2 cups ground beef
- ¼ cup tomato paste
- 1 tablespoon ground black pepper
- 3 cups of water
- 1 tablespoon olive oil
- 1 tablespoon lemon juice
- 1 tablespoon cilantro
- 1 teaspoon salt
- ¼ cup of soy sauce
- 1 teaspoon sliced garlic

Directions:

1. Place the ground beef in the pressure cooker.
2. Add the ground black pepper, cilantro, salt, and sliced garlic.

3. Sprinkle the mixture with olive oil and stir. Set the pressure cooker mode to "Sauté" the meat for 6 minutes.

4. Stir the ground meat mixture well. Add cauliflower rice and combine.

5. Add tomato paste, water, and lemon juice. Stir the mixture and close the lid. Set the pressure cooker mode to "Saute" and cook for 20 minutes.

6. When the dish is cooked, sprinkle it with the soy sauce and stir. Transfer the dish to serving bowls.

Nutrition: calories 194, fat 11.9, fiber 1.9, carbs 7, protein 15.5

Provolone Pepper Soup

Prep time: 10 minutes
Cooking time: 18 minutes
Servings: 4

Ingredients:

- 3 oz bacon, chopped
- 10 oz chicken fillet, chopped
- 3 oz Provolone cheese, grated
- 1 tablespoon cream cheese
- 1 white onion, diced
- ½ teaspoon salt
- ½ teaspoon ground black pepper
- 1 teaspoon dried parsley
- 1 garlic clove, diced
- 4 cups of water

Directions:

1. Place the chopped bacon in the instant pot and cook it for 5 minutes on sauté mode.
2. Stir it from time to time to avoid burning.
3. After this, transfer the cooked bacon in the plate and dry little with the paper towel.
4. Then add onion and diced garlic in the instant pot.

5. Sauté the vegetables for 2 minutes and add chicken and cream cheese. Stir well and sauté the ingredients for 5 minutes.

6. After this, add salt, ground black pepper, dried parsley, water, and Provolone cheese. Stir the soup mixture well.

7. Close the lid and cook the soup for 5 minutes on manual mode (high pressure). Then make a quick pressure release. Add the cooked bacon in the soup.

8. Stir the cooked soup well before serving.

Nutrition value/serving: calories 346, fat 20.7, fiber 0.7, carbs 3.8, protein 34.4

Jalapeno Garlic Soup

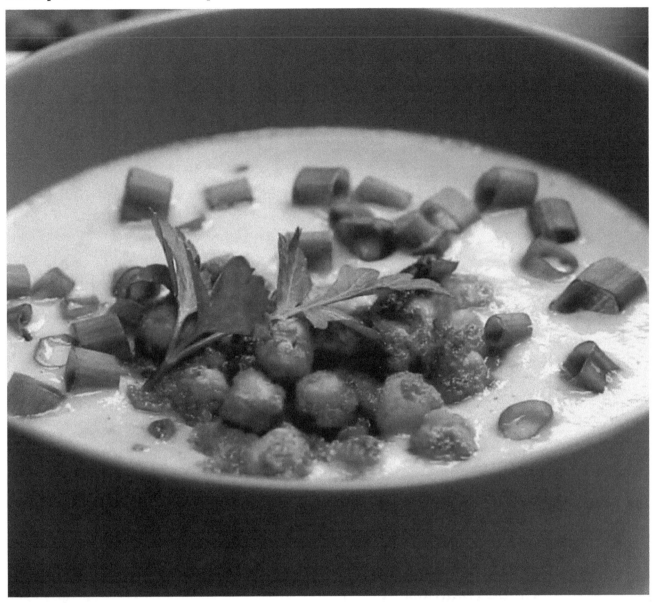

Prep time: 10 minutes

Cooking time: 20 minutes

Servings: 4

Ingredients:

- ½ cup ground pork
- 1 teaspoon garlic powder

- 1 bell pepper, diced
- 1 jalapeno pepper, sliced
- 1 teaspoon coconut oil
- 1 tomato, chopped
- ½ teaspoon salt
- 1 teaspoon thyme
- 4 cups of water

Directions:

1. Put the coconut oil in the instant pot and preheat it on Saute mode.

2. When the coconut oil starts shimmering, add bell pepper and jalapeno pepper.

3. Cook the vegetables for 1 minute and stir them.

4. Add ground pork, garlic powder, tomato, salt, and thyme.

5. Stir well and sauté the ingredients for 2 minutes.

6. Then add water and close the lid.

7. Cook the jalapeno soup for 5 minutes on Manual mode (high pressure).

8. Then allow the natural pressure release for 5 minutes.

Nutrition value/serving: calories 142, fat 9.4, fiber 0.9, carbs 3.7, protein 10.7

Eggplant Lasagna with Mozzarella

Prep time: 15 minutes

Cooking time: 10 minutes

Servings: 6

Ingredients:

- 2 eggplants, peeled, sliced
- 1 cup ground pork
- 3 tablespoons marinara sauce
- 1 white onion, diced
- 1 oz fresh basil, chopped
- ½ cup Ricotta cheese
- ½ cup Mozzarella, shredded
- ½ teaspoon dried oregano
- ¼ teaspoon salt
- 1 cup water, for cooking

Directions:

1. In the mixing bowl combine together ground pork, diced onion, basil, and dried oregano.

2. Add salt and stir the meat mixture well with the help of the spoon.

3. Line the baking pan with paper foil.

4. Then place the sliced eggplants in the baking pan to make the layer.

5. Sprinkle the eggplants with marinara sauce.

6. Top the marinara sauce with ground pork mixture.

7. Then spread the mixture with Ricotta cheese and shredded Mozzarella.

8. Cover the lasagna with foil.

9. Pour water in the instant pot and insert the trivet.

10. Place the lasagna on the trivet and close the lid.

11. Cook the lasagna for 10 minutes on manual mode (high pressure).

12. Then make a quick pressure release.

13. Cool the cooked lasagna little before serving.

Nutrition value/serving: calories 251, fat 13.5, fiber 7.2, carbs 14.9, protein 18.7

Keto Cauliflower Soup

Prep time: 15 minutes

Cooking time: 4 minutes

Servings: 2

Ingredients:

- 1 cup cauliflower, chopped
- 1 oz bacon, chopped, cooked
- 2 oz Cheddar cheese, shredded
- 2 tablespoons cream cheese
- 1 oz leek, chopped
- 1 cup of water
- ½ teaspoon salt
- ½ teaspoon cayenne pepper

Directions:

1. Pour water in the instant pot.
2. Add cauliflower, cream cheese, leek, salt, and cayenne pepper.
3. Close the lid and cook soup mixture for 4 minutes on Manual mode (high pressure).
4. Allow the natural pressure release for 10 minutes.
5. Then add cheese and stir the soup until it is melted.
6. With the help of the immersion blender, blend the soup until you get the creamy texture.

7. Then ladle the soup in the serving bowls and top with bacon.

Nutrition value/serving: calories 248, fat 19, fiber 1.6, carbs 5.7, protein 14.3

Chili Egg Soup

Prep time: 5 minutes

Cooking time: 15 minutes

Servings: 2

Ingredients:

- 2 eggs, beaten
- 2 cups chicken broth
- 1 tablespoon chives, chopped
- ½ teaspoon salt
- ½ teaspoon chili flakes

Directions:

1. Pour chicken broth in the instant pot.
2. Add chives, salt, and chili flakes.
3. Saute the liquid for 10 minutes.
4. Then add beaten eggs and stir the soup well.
5. Cook the soup for 5 minutes more.

Nutrition value/serving: calories 102, fat 5.8, fiber 0.1, carbs 1.3, protein 10.5

Beef Soup

Prep time: 10 minutes
Cooking time: 15 minutes
Servings: 6

Ingredients:
- 1 cup white cabbage, shredded
- ½ cup kale, chopped
- 11 oz beef sirloin, chopped
- ½ teaspoon salt
- 1 teaspoon dried basil
- ½ teaspoon fennel seeds
- ½ teaspoon ground black pepper
- 1 garlic clove, diced
- 1 teaspoon almond butter
- 5 cups of water

Directions:
1. Put almond butter in the instant pot and melt it on sauté mode.
2. Add white cabbage and diced garlic. Cook the vegetables for 5 minutes. Stir them occasionally.
3. Then add chopped beef sirloin, fennel seeds, ground black pepper, salt, and stir well.
4. Add basil and water.
5. Then add kale and close the lid.

6.   Cook the soup on Manual mode (high pressure) for 5 minutes.

7.   Then make a quick pressure release.

Nutrition value/serving: calories 120, fat 4.8, fiber 0.8, carbs 2.1, protein 16.7

Hot Spinach Chowder

Prep time: 10 minutes
Cooking time: 20 minutes
Servings: 4

Ingredients:

- 1 cup fresh spinach, chopped
- ½ cup heavy cream
- 4 oz bacon, chopped, cooked
- 1 teaspoon dried dill
- ½ teaspoon salt
- 4 chicken thighs, skinless, boneless, chopped
- ½ teaspoon cayenne pepper
- ½ teaspoon ground thyme
- 1 teaspoon coconut oil
- 1 teaspoon minced garlic
- 4 cups of water
- ½ cup mushrooms, chopped

Directions:

1. Put coconut oil in the instant pot and melt it on sauté mode.
2. Then add chopped chicken thighs, salt, dill, cayenne pepper, and ground thyme.
3. Stir the chicken well and sauté for 5 minutes.

4. After this, add minced garlic and chopped mushrooms. Stir well and cook for 5 minutes more.

5. Then add heavy cream and water.

6. Then add chopped spinach and bacon. Close the lid and cook the chowder on Manual mode (high pressure) for 10 minutes.

7. Then make a quick pressure release and open the lid.

8. Cool the chowder for 10-15 minutes before serving.

Nutrition value/serving: calories 249, fat 19.4, fiber 0.4, carbs 2, protein 16.4

Butternut Ginger Soup

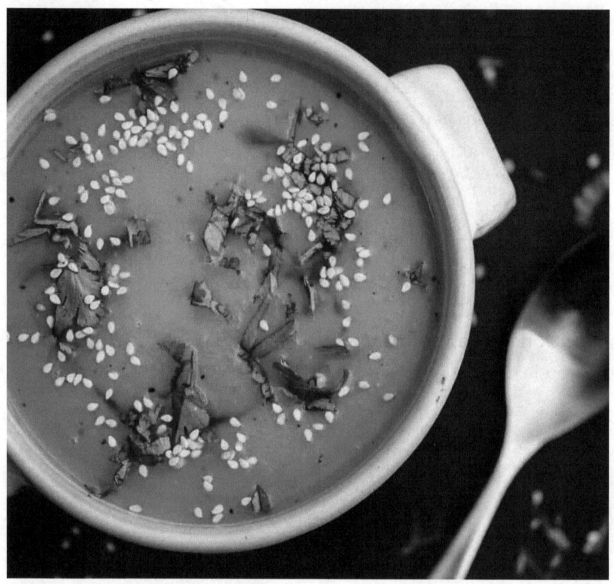

Prep time: 10 minutes

Cooking time: 25 minutes

Servings: 6

Ingredients:

- 2 cups butternut squash, chopped
- 2 garlic cloves, peeled, diced
- 1 teaspoon curry powder

- ½ teaspoon ginger, minced
- 1 white onion, diced
- 1 teaspoon salt
- 1 teaspoon ground paprika
- 1 tablespoon butter
- 5 cups chicken broth
- 2 tablespoons Ricotta cheese

Directions:

1. Melt butter in sauté mode.

2. Then add garlic and onion. Saute the vegetables until they are golden brown.

3. Then add butternut squash, ginger, salt, ground paprika, and ricotta cheese.

4. Then add curry powder and chicken broth.

5. Close the lid and cook the soup on manual mode (high pressure) for 15 minutes.

6. Then make a quick pressure release.

7. Blend the soup with the help of the immersion blender.

Nutrition value/serving: calories 87, fat 3.6, fiber 1.4, carbs 8.7, protein 5.5

Tortilla Soup

Prep time: 10 minutes
Cooking time: 30 minutes
Servings: 2

Ingredients:

- ½ Poblano pepper, chopped
- ¼ teaspoon minced garlic
- ¼ teaspoon ground coriander
- ½ cup tomatoes, canned
- 1 tablespoon dried cilantro
- ¼ teaspoon salt
- 2 cups chicken broth
- 8 oz chicken breast, skinless, boneless
- 1 tablespoon lemon juice
- 1 teaspoon butter
- ¼ cup Cheddar cheese, shredded
- 2 low carb tortillas, chopped

Directions:

1. Melt butter in sauté mode.
2. When the butter is melted, add chopped Poblano pepper, minced garlic, ground coriander, and dried cilantro.
3. Add chicken breast and cook the ingredients for 10 minutes. Stir them from time to time.

4. After this, add canned tomatoes, salt, and chicken broth.

5. Close the lid and cook the soup on manual mode (high pressure) for 15 minutes.

6. Then make a quick pressure release and open the lid.

7. Add lemon juice and sauté the soup for 5 minutes more.

8. Ladle the soup into the bowls and top with Cheddar cheese and chopped low carb tortillas.

Nutrition value/serving: calories 336, fat 13, fiber 8.3, carbs 16.1, protein 36.2

Steak Zucchini Soup

Prep time: 10 minutes
Cooking time: 25 minutes
Servings: 4

Ingredients:

- ½ teaspoon minced ginger
- ¼ teaspoon minced garlic
- 1 teaspoon coconut oil
- 10 oz beef sirloin steak, chopped
- ½ cup cremini mushrooms, sliced
- 4 cups chicken broth
- ½ teaspoon salt
- 1 zucchini, trimmed
- 1 teaspoon chives, chopped

Directions:

1.   Heat up instant pot on sauté mode.
2.   Toss coconut oil and melt it.
3.   Then add minced ginger and minced garlic. Stir well and add chopped steak.
4.   Sauté the mixture for 5 minutes.
5.   Meanwhile, with the help of the spiralizer make the zucchini noodles.
6.   Add mushrooms in the beef mixture. Then sprinkle it with salt.

7.   Add chicken broth and cook the soup on Manual mode (high pressure) for 12 minutes.

8.   Then make a quick pressure release and open the lid.

9.   Add spiralized noodles and stir the soup. Let it rest for 5 minutes.

10.   Top the cooked soup with chives.

Nutrition value/serving: calories 191, fat 7, fiber 0.6, carbs 3.2, protein 27.2

Chili Meat

Prep time: 10 minutes
Cooking time: 3 hours 5 minutes
Servings: 2

Ingredients:

- 9 oz pork shoulder, chopped
- ½ cup salsa Verde
- 1 teaspoon sesame oil
- ½ cup chicken broth
- ¼ teaspoon cayenne pepper
- ¼ teaspoon salt

Directions:

1. Pour sesame oil in the instant pot and preheat it on sauté mode for 3 minutes.
2. Meanwhile, mix up together pork shoulder, cayenne pepper, and salt.
3. Add the pork shoulder in the hot oil and sauté the meat for 2 minutes.
4. Then stir it with the help of the spatula and add chicken broth and salsa Verde.
5. Close the lid.
6. Cook the meal on manual (low pressure) for 3 hours.
7. When the time is over, shred the meat.

Nutrition value/serving: calories 418, fat 30.1, fiber 0.3, carbs 2.9, protein 31.7

Garlic Taco Soup

Prep time: 10 minutes
Cooking time: 25 minutes
Servings: 5

Ingredients:

- 2 cups ground beef
- 1 teaspoon onion powder
- 1 teaspoon taco seasonings
- 1 garlic clove, diced
- 1 teaspoon chili flakes
- 1 teaspoon ground cumin
- 1 tablespoon tomato paste
- ½ cup heavy cream
- 5 cups of water
- 1 teaspoon coconut oil
- 1 tablespoon cream cheese
- 1 jalapeno pepper, sliced

Directions:

1. Toss the coconut oil in the instant pot and melt it on sauté mode.
2. Add ground beef and onion powder.
3. After this, add taco seasonings and diced garlic. Mix up the ingredients well.

4.   Then sprinkle the meat mixture with chili flakes and ground cumin.

5.   Saute the ground beef for 10 minutes. Mix it up with the help of the spatula every 3 minutes.

6.   Then add tomato paste, heavy cream, and water.

7.   Add sliced jalapeno pepper and close the lid.

8.   Cook the soup on Manual (high pressure) for 10 minutes.

9.   Then allow the natural pressure release for 10 minutes and ladle the soup into the bowls.

Nutrition value/serving: calories 170, fat 12.7, fiber 0.3, carbs 2.4, protein 11.2

Chicken Chipotle Soup

Prep time: 10 minutes
Cooking time: 32 minutes
Servings: 4

Ingredients:

- 1-pound chicken fillet
- ½ white onion, chopped
- 1 bell pepper, chopped
- 1 jalapeno pepper, chopped
- 1 tablespoon avocado oil
- 1 tablespoon tomato paste
- 1 teaspoon apple cider vinegar
- 1 teaspoon chipotle pepper
- ½ teaspoon garlic powder
- ½ teaspoon ground cumin
- ½ teaspoon ground coriander
- ½ teaspoon ground paprika
- 1/3 teaspoon salt
- 1 teaspoon dried oregano
- 4 cups of water

Directions:

1. Pour avocado oil in the instant pot.
2. Add white onion, bell pepper, and jalapeno pepper.
3. Saute the vegetables on sauté mode for 5 minutes.

4. Meanwhile, in the shallow bowl combine together garlic powder, cumin, coriander, paprika, salt, and dried oregano.

5. Add the spices in the vegetables.

6. Then add tomato paste, chipotle pepper, and apple cider vinegar.

7. Add water and chicken fillet.

8. Close the lid and cook enchilada soup on Manual mode (high pressure) for 25 minutes.

9. Then make a quick pressure release and open the lid.

10. With the help of 2 forks shred the chicken fillet and stir the soup.

Nutrition value/serving: calories 244, fat 9.1, fiber 1.4, carbs 5.5, protein 33.7

Creamy Cheddar Soup

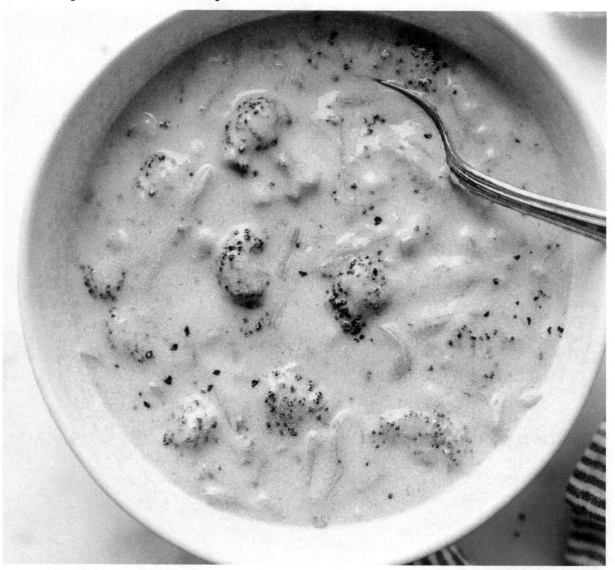

Prep time: 10 minutes

Cooking time: 15 minutes

Servings: 2

Ingredients:

- 1 tablespoon cream cheese
- 1 oz bacon, chopped, cooked
- 2 oz Cheddar cheese, shredded

- 2 cups cauliflower, chopped
- ½ teaspoon salt
- 1 teaspoon dried oregano
- 2 cups chicken broth
- ½ teaspoon ground nutmeg
- ½ medium white onion, diced

Directions:

1. Place onion and cream cheese in the instant pot.

2. Cook the ingredients on sauté mode until onion is light brown.

3. Then add chopped cauliflower, salt, dried oregano, and ground nutmeg.

4. Cook the vegetables for 3 minutes.

5. Then stir them well and add chicken broth.

6. Cook the soup on Manual (High pressure) for 4 minutes.

7. Then make a quick pressure release and open the lid.

8. With the help of immersion blender, blend the soup until smooth.

9. Ladle the soup in the bowls and top with Cheddar cheese and cook bacon.

Nutrition value/serving: calories 286, fat 18.8, fiber 3.2, carbs 9.7, protein 19.9

Sausage Soup

Prep time: 10 minutes
Cooking time: 17 minutes
Servings: 4

Ingredients:

- 3 cups of water
- 9 oz sausages, chopped
- 2 oz Parmesan
- ½ cup heavy cream
- 2 cups kale, chopped
- ½ teaspoon ground black pepper
- ¼ onion, diced
- 1 teaspoon dried basil
- 1 tablespoon olive oil

Directions:

1. Pour olive oil in the instant pot and add the onion.
2. Saute the onion for 3 minutes.
3. Then stir well and add sausages. Mix up well and cook them for 3 minutes.
4. After this, add water, kale, basil, and ground black pepper.
5. Saute the mixture for 8 minutes.
6. Then add heavy cream and Parmesan.

7.   Close the lid and cook the soup on manual mode (high pressure) for 3 minutes. Then make a quick pressure release.

8.   Let the cooked kale soup cool for 10-15 minutes before serving.

Nutrition value/serving: calories 364, fat 30.2, fiber 0.7, carbs 5.3, protein 18.4

Bone Broth Soup

Prep time: 7 minutes
Cooking time: 10 minutes
Servings: 2

Ingredients:

- 1 eggplant, trimmed, chopped
- 2 cups bone broth
- ¼ cup carrot, grated
- 1 tablespoon butter
- ½ teaspoon salt
- 1 teaspoon dried dill

Directions:

1.   In the mixing bowl combine together eggplants and salt. Leave the vegetables for 5 minutes.
2.   Meanwhile, toss the butter in the instant pot and melt it on sauté mode.
3.   Add grated carrot and cook it for 2 minutes.
4.   Meanwhile, dry the eggplants.
5.   Add them in the carrot and stir. Sprinkle the vegetables with dried dill.
6.   Then add bone broth and close the lid.
7.   Cook the soup for 5 minutes on Manual mode (high pressure). Then make a quick pressure release.

Nutrition value/serving: calories 200, fat 6.2, fiber 8.5, carbs 15.1, protein 22.5

Celery Chicken Soup

Prep time: 10 minutes

Cooking time: 15 minutes

Servings: 5

Ingredients:
- 1 white onion, diced
- ½ cup celery stalk, chopped
- ½ teaspoon minced garlic
- 1 teaspoon olive oil
- 1-pound chicken breast, cooked, shredded
- 4 cups chicken broth
- 1 tablespoon buffalo sauce

Directions:
1. In the instant pot bowl mix up together onion, minced garlic, and olive oil.
2. Cook the ingredients on sauté mode for 4 minutes.
3. Then stir them well and add shredded chicken breast.
4. Add chicken broth and buffalo sauce. Mix up well.
5. Cook the soup on soup mode for 10 minutes.

Nutrition value/serving: calories 154, fat 4.3, fiber 0.7, carbs 3.4, protein 23.4

Cream & Vegetable Stew

Prep time: 10 minutes
Cooking time: 25 minutes
Servings: 2

Ingredients:

- 4 oz sausages, chopped
- ½ cup savoy cabbage, chopped
- 2 oz turnip, chopped
- ¼ cup bok choy, chopped
- 1 teaspoon ground cumin
- ¼ teaspoon fennel seeds
- ½ cup heavy cream
- ½ teaspoon salt
- 1 teaspoon butter

Directions:

1. Preheat the instant pot on sauté mode for 2 minutes.

2. Toss the butter inside and melt it.

3. After this, add sausages and cook them for 5 minutes on sauté mode. Stir them from time to time.

4. Then add salt, fennel seeds, ground cumin, and heavy cream.

5. Add savoy cabbage, turnip, and bok choy. Stir the stew well.

6. Cook the stew on stew mode for 15 minutes.

Nutrition value/serving: calories 331, fat 29.4, fiber 1.3, carbs 4.5, protein 12.5

Broccoli Lunch Bowl

Prep time: 10 minutes
Cooking time: 25 minutes
Servings: 2

Ingredients:
- ½ cup broccoli, chopped
- 8 oz chicken fillet, chopped
- 1 green bell pepper, chopped
- 1 teaspoon ground black pepper
- ½ teaspoon dried cilantro
- 1 cup chicken broth
- ½ teaspoon salt
- ½ teaspoon almond butter

Directions:
1. Place almond butter, bell pepper, and broccoli in the instant pot.
2. Cook the ingredients on sauté mode for 5 minutes. Stir them with the help of the spatula from time to time.
3. After this, add chopped chicken fillet, ground black pepper, salt, and cilantro.
4. Add chicken broth and mix up the meal well.
5. Close the lid and cook it on stew mode for 20 minutes.

6. When the meal is cooked, let it rest for 10 minutes before serving.

Nutrition value/serving: calories 289, fat 11.6, fiber 2.1, carbs 7.9, protein 37.4

Cabbage Salad

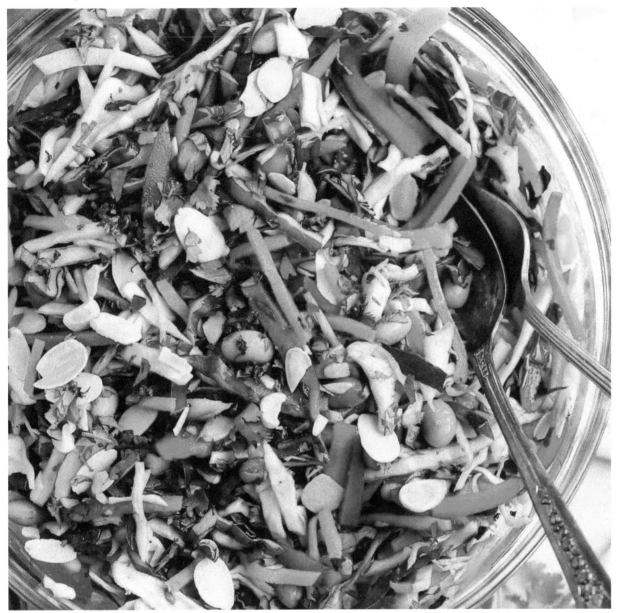

Prep time: 10 minutes

Cooking time: 21 minutes

Servings: 4

Ingredients:

- 1-pound chicken breast, skinless, boneless
- 1 avocado, pitted, peeled

- 4 eggs
- 1 cup lettuce, chopped
- 1 tablespoon lemon juice
- ¼ teaspoon salt
- ½ teaspoon white pepper
- ½ cup white cabbage, shredded
- 4 oz Feta cheese, crumbled
- 1 tablespoon coconut oil
- ½ teaspoon chili flakes
- 1 tablespoon heavy cream
- 1 tablespoon apple cider vinegar
- ½ teaspoon garlic powder
- 1 cup water, for cooking

Directions:

1. Pour water and insert the trivet in the instant pot.

2. Place the eggs on the trivet and close the lid.

3. Cook them in manual mode (high pressure) for 5 minutes. Then make a quick pressure release.

4. Cool the eggs in ice water. Then peel the eggs.

5. Cut the eggs and avocado into the wedges.

6. After this, rub the chicken breast with lemon juice, salt, and coconut oil.

7. Place the chicken breast in the instant pot and cook it on sauté mode for 7 minutes from each side. The cooked chicken should be light brown.

8. Make the sauce: whisk together chili flakes, olive oil, heavy cream, apple cider vinegar, and garlic powder.

9. In the big salad bowl combine together lettuce, eggs, avocado, white pepper, white cabbage, and crumbled feta.

10. Chop the cooked chicken roughly and add in the salad. Shake the salad well.

11. Then sprinkle the cooked cobb salad with sauce.

Nutrition value/serving: calories 417, fat 27.9, fiber 3.8, carbs 7.4, protein 34.9

Cucumber and Lobster Salad

Prep time: 10 minutes
Cooking time: 4 minutes
Servings: 4

Ingredients:

- 4 lobster tails, peeled
- 1 teaspoon avocado oil
- ¼ teaspoon salt
- 2 cucumbers, chopped
- ¼ cup whipped cream
- 1 tablespoon apple cider vinegar
- 1 teaspoon dried dill
- ½ cup celery stalk, chopped
- 1 cup water, for cooking

Directions:

1. Pour water and insert the trivet in the instant pot.

2. Arrange the lobster tails on the trivet and cook them on Manual mode (high pressure) for 4 minutes. Then make a quick pressure release.

3. Cool the cooked lobster tails little and chop them roughly.

4. Place the chopped lobster tails in the salad bowl.

5. Add cucumbers, dried ill, and celery stalk.

6.   After this, make the salad sauce: in the shallow bowl combine together salt, avocado oil, whipped cream, dill, and apple cider vinegar.

7.   Sprinkle the salad with sauce and mix up it well with the help of 2 spoons.

Nutrition value/serving: calories 139, fat 3.7, fiber 1, carbs 6.3, protein 1.3

Italian Salad

Prep time: 5 minutes
Cooking time: 5 minutes
Servings: 2

Ingredients:

- 8 oz shrimps, peeled
- 1 teaspoon Italian seasonings
- 1 teaspoon olive oil
- ½ cup cherry tomatoes, halved
- ¼ teaspoon chili flakes
- ½ teaspoon coconut oil

Directions:

1. Toss coconut oil in the instant pot.
2. Melt it on sauté mode and add peeled shrimps.
3. Cook the shrimps for 1 minute from each side.
4. Then place the shrimps in the bowl.
5. Add chili flakes, Italian seasonings, halved cherry tomatoes, and olive oil.
6. Shake the salad before serving.

Nutrition value/serving: calories 173, fat 5.5, fiber 0.5, carbs 3.5, protein 26.2

Egg Salad and Cheddar with Dill

Prep time: 15 minutes

Cooking time: 4 minutes

Servings: 3

Ingredients:

- 3 eggs
- 2 tablespoons cream cheese
- 1 tablespoon dried dill
- ½ cup Cheddar cheese, shredded
- ¼ teaspoon minced garlic
- 1 cup water, for cooking

Directions:

1. Pour water and insert rack in the instant pot.
2. Place the eggs in the instant pot, close the lid and cook them for 4 minutes on Manual mode (high pressure). Then make a quick pressure release.
3. Cool the eggs in cold water for 10 minutes.
4. After this, peel the eggs and grate them.
5. In the mixing bowl combine together grated eggs, shredded cheese, minced garlic, dill, and cream cheese.
6. Mix up the salad well.

Nutrition value/serving: calories 165, fat 13, fiber 0.1, carbs 1.4, protein 11

Cream Cheese Salad

Prep time: 10 minutes
Cooking time: 2 minutes
Servings: 2

Ingredients:

- 10 oz crab meat
- 1 tablespoon sour cream
- 1 tablespoon cream
- ¼ teaspoon minced garlic
- 1 tablespoon cream cheese
- ½ teaspoon lime juice
- ½ red onion, diced
- ¼ cup fresh cilantro, chopped
- ¼ cup fresh spinach, chopped
- ¼ teaspoon salt
- ¼ teaspoon ground cumin
- 1 cup water, for cooking

Directions:

1. Pour water in the instant pot.

2. Line the trivet with the paper foil and insert the instant pot.

3. Place the crab meat on the trivet and cook it on Manual mode (high pressure) for 2 minutes. Then make a

quick pressure release and remove the crab meat from the instant pot.

4. Chop it and place it in the salad bowl.
5. Add diced onion, spinach, and cilantro.
6. In the shallow bowl make the salad dressing: whisk together sour cream, cream, minced garlic, cream cheese, and lime juice.
7. Then add salt and ground cumin.
8. Add the dressing in the salad and stir it well.

Nutrition value/serving: calories 175, fat 6, fiber 0.8, carbs 6.4, protein 18.9

Chicken Paprika

Prep time: 10 minutes
Cooking time: 25 minutes
Servings: 2

Ingredients:

- 2 chicken thighs, skinless, boneless
- 2 tablespoons ground paprika
- 1 tablespoon almond meal
- 1 teaspoon tomato paste
- ½ teaspoon dried celery root
- ½ cup heavy cream
- 1 tablespoon butter
- ½ teaspoon salt
- ½ teaspoon white pepper
- ¼ teaspoon ground nutmeg
- 1 tablespoon lemon juice

Directions:

1. Melt butter in sauté mode.
2. Meanwhile, rub the chicken thighs with salt and white pepper.
3. Cook the chicken thighs on sauté mode for 4 minutes from each side.
4. Meanwhile, in the mixing bowl combine together almond meal, dried celery root, and ground nutmeg.

5. In the separated bowl combine together heavy cream, tomato paste, and lemon juice.

6. Pour the heavy cream liquid in the chicken.

7. Then add almond meal mixture and stir gently.

8. Cook the meal on meat mode for 15 minutes.

Nutrition value/serving: calories 476, fat 30.3, fiber 3.3, carbs 6.5, protein 44.8

Cauliflower and Eggs Salad

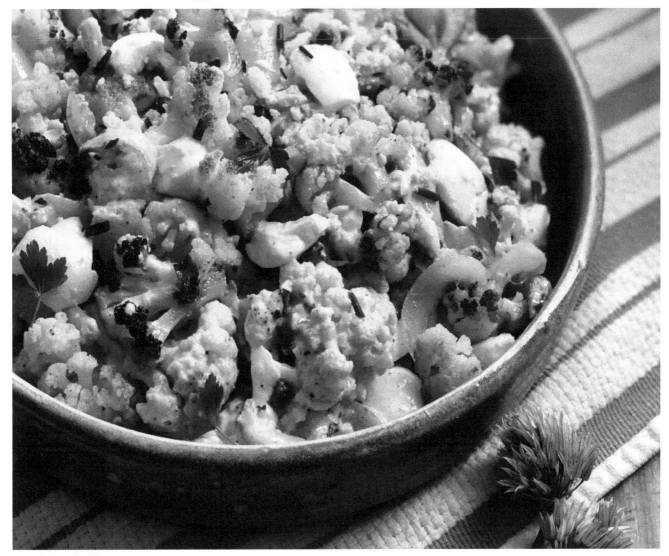

Prep time: 10 minutes

Cooking time: 9 minutes

Servings: 2

Ingredients:

- 1 cup cauliflower, chopped
- 2 eggs
- 1/3 teaspoon salt
- ½ cup purple cabbage, shredded

- 1 tablespoon lemon juice
- 1 tablespoon cream cheese
- 4 oz bacon, chopped, cooked
- 1 cup water, for cooking

Directions:

1.   Pour water and insert the trivet in the instant pot.

2.   Place the eggs on the trivet and cook them on manual mode (high pressure) for 5 minutes. Then make a quick pressure release.

3.   Cool the eggs.

4.   Place the cauliflower on the trivet and cook on steam mode for 4 minutes. Make a quick pressure release.

5.   Peel and chop the eggs.

6.   Place the eggs in the mixing bowl.

7.   Add cooked cauliflower, salt, shredded purple cabbage, lemon juice, cream cheese, and bacon.

8.   Mix up the salad.

Nutrition value/serving: calories 406, fat 29.9, fiber 1.7, carbs 5.1, protein 28.2

Lemon Radish Salad

Prep time: 10 minutes
Cooking time: 11 minutes
Servings: 4

Ingredients:
- 3 cups radish, sliced
- 7 oz chicken fillet, chopped
- 1 tablespoon lemon juice
- 1 teaspoon olive oil
- ¼ teaspoon salt
- 1 teaspoon butter
- 1 tablespoon dried parsley
- ½ teaspoon sesame oil

Directions:
1. Mix up together chopped chicken fillet with lemon juice, olive oil, and salt.
2. Place the chicken in the instant pot and cook it on sauté mode for 3 minutes from each side.
3. Then add radish and butter, and sauté the ingredients for 5 minutes.
4. Transfer the cooked salad in the bowl.
5. Add dried parsley and sesame oil. Mix up the salad.

Nutrition value/serving: calories 133, fat 6.5, fiber 1.4, carbs 3.1, protein 15

Cream Chicken

Prep time: 10 minutes
Cooking time: 10 minutes
Servings: 4

Ingredients:

- 1-pound chicken breast
- 1 teaspoon salt
- 1 teaspoon garlic powder
- ½ teaspoon ground black pepper
- 1 teaspoon sesame oil
- ½ cup chicken broth
- 2 tablespoons cream cheese
- ½ teaspoon ground cumin
- ½ teaspoon ground coriander
- ½ teaspoon onion powder
- ½ teaspoon chives

Directions:

1. Cut the chicken breast into 4 servings.
2. Then sprinkle the chicken with salt, garlic powder, sesame oil, and ground black pepper.
3. Place the chicken in the instant pot and cook it on sauté mode for 2 minutes from each side.
4. Then add chicken broth and cream cheese.

5.   Sprinkle the ingredients with ground cumin, coriander, onion powder, and chives.

6.   Stir the chicken with the help of the spatula and close the lid.

7.   Cook the crack chicken on poultry mode for 5 minutes.

Nutrition value/serving: calories 167, fat 6, fiber 0.2, carbs 1.3, protein 25.3

Salsa Chicken

Prep time: 15 minutes
Cooking time: 17 minutes
Servings: 2

Ingredients:

- ¼ cup hot salsa
- 10 oz chicken breast, skinless, boneless
- 1 teaspoon taco seasoning
- ¼ teaspoon salt
- ¼ teaspoon chili flakes
- 1 tablespoon cream cheese
- ¼ cup chicken broth

Directions:

1. Place the chicken breast in the instant pot.
2. Sprinkle the poultry with taco seasoning, salt, and chili flakes.
3. Then add cream cheese, salsa, and chicken broth.
4. Close and seal the lid.
5. Cook the meal on manual mode (high pressure) for 17 minutes.
6. Then allow the natural pressure release for 10 minutes and shred the chicken.
7. Serve the shredded chicken with hot sauce from the instant pot.

Nutrition value/serving: calories 198, fat 5.5, fiber 0.5, carbs 3.3, protein 31.5

Onion Carnitas

Prep time: 10 minutes
Cooking time: 30 minutes
Servings: 4

Ingredients:

- 13 oz pork butt, chopped
- ¼ cup white onion, diced
- 1 teaspoon ghee
- ½ teaspoon garlic powder
- 1 tablespoon lemon juice
- ¼ teaspoon grated lemon zest
- ½ teaspoon chipotle powder
- 1 cup of water
- ½ teaspoon salt
- 1 cup lettuce leaves

Directions:

1. Put pork butt, white onion, ghee, garlic powder, lemon juice, grated lemon zest, and chipotle powder in the instant pot.

2. Saute the ingredients for 5 minutes.

3. Then mix up the meat mixture with the help of the spatula and add salt and water.

4. Close and seal the lid and cook ingredients on manual mode (high pressure) for 25 minutes.

5.   When the time is over, make a quick pressure release and open the lid.

6.   Shred the cooked pork with the help of the fork.

7.   Then fill the lettuce leaves with shredded pork.

Nutrition value/serving: calories 194 fat 7.3, fiber 0.3, carbs 1.4, protein 28.9

Smoky Paprika Pork

Prep time: 10 minutes
Cooking time: 20 minutes
Servings: 4

Ingredients:

- 1-pound pork loin
- 1 teaspoon smoked paprika
- ½ teaspoon liquid smoke
- ½ teaspoon ground coriander
- ½ teaspoon salt
- 1 teaspoon onion powder
- 1 teaspoon tomato paste
- 1 cup chicken broth

Directions:

1. Put the pork loin in the instant pot.

2. Add smoked paprika, liquid smoke, ground coriander, salt, onion powder, tomato paste, and chicken broth.

3. Close the lid and cook the pork on manual mode (high pressure) for 20 minutes.

4. When the time is over, make a quick pressure release and open the lid.

5. Remove the pork loin from the instant pot and shred it.

6. Place the cooked pulled pork in the bowl and sprinkle it with ½ part of liquid from the instant pot.

Nutrition value/serving: calories 233, fat 8, fiber 0.3, carbs 1.3, protein 36.7

Chicken Coconut Soup

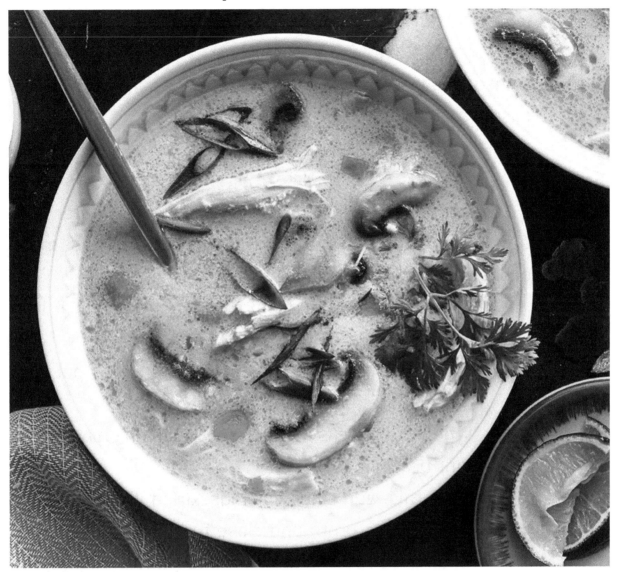

Prep time: 10 minutes

Cooking time: 25 minutes

Servings: 4

Ingredients:

- 4 cups chicken broth
- 4 chicken wings
- ½ onion, diced

- 1 tablespoon dried dill
- ½ teaspoon salt
- ¼ cup coconut flour
- 2 tablespoons water
- 1 teaspoon ghee

Directions:

1. In the mixing bowl combine together water and coconut flour. Knead the non-sticky dough. Add more coconut flour if the dough is sticky.

2. Then make the log from the dough and cut it into pieces.

3. After this, place the ghee in the instant pot and preheat it on sauté mode.

4. When the ghee is melted, add diced onion and cook it until light brown.

5. After this, add chicken wings, dried ill, and salt.

6. Add chicken broth and close the lid.

7. Cook the soup on manual mode (high pressure) for 10 minutes. Then make a quick pressure release.

8. Open the lid and add prepared dough pieces (dumplings). Sauté the soup for 5 minutes more.

Nutrition value/serving: calories 179, fat 9.5, fiber 3.5, carbs 10.8, protein 11.9

Zoodle Soup

Prep time: 10 minutes
Cooking time: 25 minutes
Servings: 2

Ingredients:

- 2 cups chicken broth
- ½ teaspoon salt
- ½ teaspoon chili flakes
- 1 teaspoon dried oregano
- 1 teaspoon butter
- 8 oz chicken tenderloins
- 1 zucchini, spiralized

Directions:

1. Melt the butter in sauté mode.
2. Then add chicken tenderloins.
3. Sprinkle them with chili flakes, dried oregano, and salt.
4. Cook the chicken for 3 minutes.
5. Then add chicken broth and close the lid.
6. Cook the soup on manual mode (high pressure) for 10 minutes.
7. When the time is over, make a quick pressure release and open the lid.

8. Add spiralized zucchini and stir the soup. Leave it to rest for 10 minutes.

Nutrition value/serving: calories 170, fat 4.1, fiber 1.4, carbs 4.7, protein 29.1

Spinach and Beef Soup

Prep time: 10 minutes
Cooking time: 23 minutes
Servings: 3

Ingredients:

- 2 cups spinach, chopped
- 2 cups beef broth
- 7 oz sausages, chopped
- 1 teaspoon ghee
- ½ teaspoon salt
- ½ teaspoon ground cumin
- ½ teaspoon ground coriander
- ½ teaspoon dried celery
- ½ teaspoon onion powder
- 2 bell peppers, chopped

Directions:

1. Preheat the instant pot on sauté mode and place ghee inside.
2. Melt it and add sausages.
3. Cook the sausages for 10 minutes. Stir them from time to time with the help of the spatula.
4. After this, sprinkle the sausages with salt, ground cumin, coriander, dried celery, and onion powder.
5. Add beef broth and bell peppers.

6. Close and seal the lid.

7. Cook the soup on manual mode (high pressure) for 5 minutes.

8. Then make a quick pressure release and open the lid.

9. Stir the soup and add spinach.

10. Cook the soup for 5 minutes more on sauté mode.

Nutrition value/serving: calories 295, fat 21.4, fiber 1.6, carbs 7.8, protein 17.6

Jalapeno and Cream Soup

Prep time: 10 minutes
Cooking time: 20 minutes
Servings: 4

Ingredients:

- ¼ cup cream cheese
- 12 oz chicken fillet
- ½ teaspoon taco seasonings
- 2 bell peppers, chopped
- ½ cup canned tomatoes
- 3 cups beef broth
- ½ teaspoon salt
- ¼ cup heavy cream
- 1 jalapeno pepper, sliced
- 1 chili pepper, sliced
- 1 tablespoon butter
- ½ teaspoon minced garlic

Directions:

1. Melt the butter in sauté mode and add chicken fillet.

2. Sprinkle it with taco seasonings, salt, and minced garlic.

3. Cook it for 4 minutes from each side.

4.   After this, add cream cheese, canned tomatoes, cream, and bell peppers.

5.   Close the lid and cook the soup on manual mode (high pressure) for 10 minutes.

6.   Then make a quick pressure release and open the lid.

7.   Shred the chicken with the help of the fork.

8.   Add sliced chili pepper and jalapeno pepper in the soup and cook it on sauté mode for 5 minutes more.

Nutrition value/serving: calories 320, fat 18.3, fiber 1.2, carbs 7.6, protein 30.4

Kalua Smoked Chicken

Prep time: 15 minutes
Cooking time: 15 minutes
Servings: 3

Ingredients:

- 3 bacon slices
- ¼ teaspoon salt
- ¼ teaspoon of liquid smoked
- 6 chicken thighs, skinless, boneless
- 1/3 cup water

Directions:

1. Place the bacon at the bottom of the instant pot bowl.

2. Sprinkle the chicken thighs with salt and liquid smoker and place over the bacon.

3. Then add water, close and seal the lid.

4. Cook the chicken on manual mode (high pressure) for 15 minutes.

5. When the time is over, allow the natural pressure release and transfer the chicken tights on the chopping board.

6. Shred the chicken and transfer it in the serving plates.

7. Chop the cooked bacon.

8.   Sprinkle the cooked chicken with instant pot liquid and cooked bacon.

Nutrition value/serving: calories 363, fat 21.9, fiber 0, carbs 0.3, protein 45

Celery and Beef Chili

Prep time: 5 minutes

Cooking time: 25 minutes

Servings: 2

Ingredients:

- 1 cup ground beef
- ¼ cup celery stalk, chopped
- ¼ onion, chopped
- 1 teaspoon chili powder
- ¼ teaspoon salt
- 1 tablespoon tomato paste
- 1 cup chicken stock
- 1 teaspoon butter
- ½ teaspoon smoked paprika
- 1 tablespoon salsa

Directions:

1. Put the butter in the instant pot bowl.

2. Add ground beef and cook it on sauté mode for 5 minutes.

3. Then stir the ground beef and sprinkle it with chili powder, salt, smoked paprika, and salsa.

4. Add tomato paste, onion, and celery stalk.

5. Add chicken stock.

6. Close the lid and cook chili on stew mode for 20 minutes.

Nutrition value/serving: calories 173, fat 10.7, fiber 1.6, carbs 5.1, protein 14.3

Spicy Clam Chowder

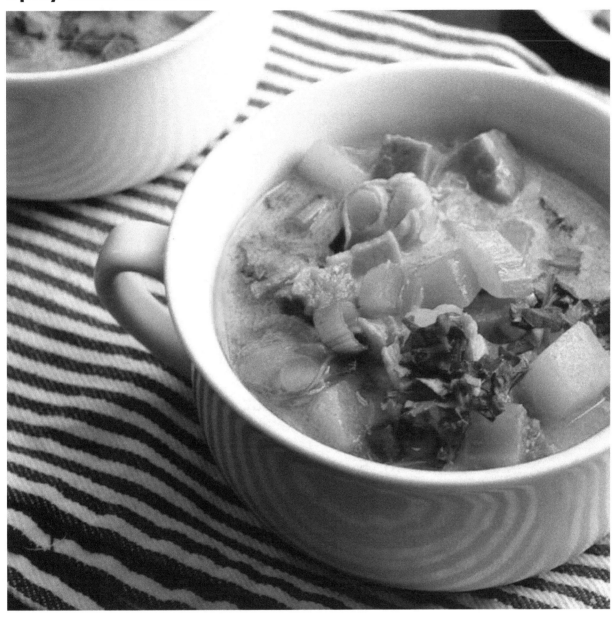

Prep time: 10 minutes

Cooking time: 22 minutes

Servings: 5

Ingredients:

- 8 oz clams, canned
- ¼ cup clam juice

- ½ cup celery stalk, chopped
- 2 cups cauliflower, chopped
- 2 oz bacon, chopped
- ½ white onion, diced
- ½ teaspoon ground coriander
- ½ teaspoon ground thyme
- ¼ teaspoon salt
- ¼ teaspoon ground black pepper
- ½ teaspoon coconut oil
- 3 cups of water
- ½ cup heavy cream

Directions:

1.   Set sauté mode and put the bacon in the instant pot.

2.   Cook it for 5 minutes. Stir it from time to time.

3.   After this, transfer the cooked bacon on the plate.

4.   Put coconut oil in the instant pot and add the onion. Cook it for 4 minutes or until it is light brown.

5.   Then add cauliflower, celery stalk, water, ad clam juice.

6.   Close and seal the lid and cook the chowder for 5 minutes on Manual mode (high pressure).

7.   When the time is over, make a quick pressure release and open the lid.

8.   Blend the mixture with the help of the immersion blender.

9.   Then add canned clams, ground coriander, thyme, salt, ground black pepper, and heavy cream.

10.   Cook the chowder on sauté mode for 5 minutes more.

11.   Ladle the cooked chowder in the bowls and sprinkle with bacon.

Nutrition value/serving: calories 145, fat 9.8, fiber 1.7, carbs 9, protein 5.8

Parsley Meatloaf

Prep time: 15 minutes
Cooking time: 30 minutes
Servings: 7

Ingredients:
- 2 cups ground beef
- 1 tablespoon parsley, chopped
- 1 teaspoon minced garlic
- 1 egg, beaten
- 1 teaspoon chili powder
- 2 oz Parmesan, grated
- 1 teaspoon butter, melted
- 1 tablespoon pork rinds
- 1 cup water, for cooking

Directions:
1. In the big bowl combine together ground beef, parsley, minced garlic, egg, chili powder, Parmesan, and pork rinds.
2. Mix up the mixture until smooth.
3. After this, pour water and insert the rack in the instant pot.
4. Line the rack with foil and place the ground beef mixture on it.

5.   Make the shape of the meatloaf with the help of the fingertips.

6.   Then brush the surface of meatloaf with butter and close the lid.

7.   Cook the meatloaf for 30 minutes on Manual mode (high pressure).

8.   Then make a quick pressure release.

9.   Cool the meatloaf well.

Nutrition value/serving: calories 127, fat 8.4, fiber 0.2, carbs 0.7, protein 12.2

Pepper Rosemary Chops

Prep time: 10 minutes
Cooking time: 25 minutes
Servings: 4

Ingredients:

- 16 oz pork chops
- ½ teaspoon ground black pepper
- ½ teaspoon salt
- ½ teaspoon chili flakes
- ¼ teaspoon cayenne pepper
- 1 tablespoon sesame oil
- 1 teaspoon lemon juice
- ½ teaspoon dried rosemary
- 1 cup water, for cooking

Directions:

1. In the bowl combine together salt, ground black pepper, chili flakes, cayenne pepper, sesame oil, lemon juice, and dried rosemary.

2. Rub the pork chops with oily mixture and wrap in the foil.

3. Pour water and insert the trivet in the instant pot.

4. Place the wrapped pork chops in the instant pot and cook on manual mode (high pressure) for 25 minutes.

5. When the time is over, make a quick pressure release.

Nutrition value/serving: calories 395, fat 31.6, fiber 0.2, carbs 0.4, protein 25.5

Meat & Turmeric Bowl

Prep time: 10 minutes
Cooking time: 18 minutes
Servings: 4

Ingredients:

- 1 cup ground pork
- 2 cups collard greens, chopped
- 1 tablespoon butter
- ½ teaspoon salt
- 1 teaspoon minced garlic
- 1 teaspoon ground paprika
- 1 teaspoon ground turmeric
- ¼ cup chicken broth

Directions:

1. Melt the butter in sauté mode and add ground pork.
2. Sprinkle it with salt, minced garlic, ground paprika, and ground turmeric.
3. Cook the ground pork on sauté mode for 10 minutes. Stir it from time to time to avoid burning.
4. After this, add collard greens and chicken broth.
5. Cook the meal on manual mode (high pressure) for 5 minutes.
6. When the time is finished, make a quick pressure release.

7. Mix up the cooked meal well before serving.

Nutrition value/serving: calories 271, fat 19.5, fiber 1.1, carbs 2.2, protein 21.1

Spinach Mix

Prep time: 5 minutes

Cooking time: 10 minutes

Servings: 4

Ingredients:

- 1-pound spinach, chopped
- 2 tablespoons ghee
- 1 teaspoon garam masala
- ½ teaspoon ground coriander
- 1 teaspoon salt
- ½ teaspoon ground thyme
- ½ teaspoon cayenne pepper
- ½ teaspoon ground turmeric
- 1 teaspoon minced garlic
- ¼ cup of water

Directions:

1. Place ghee in the instant pot and melt it on sauté mode.

2. After this, add garam masala, ground coriander, salt, thyme, cayenne pepper, turmeric, and minced garlic.

3. Stir the mixture and cook it for 1 minute.

4. Then add spinach and water. Mix up the greens well with the help of the spatula.

5. Close the lid and cook the meal on sauté mode for 5 minutes.

6.   Switch off the instant pot.

7.   Open the lid and blend the spinach until you get a smooth puree.

8.   Place the spinach saag in the serving plates.

Nutrition value/serving: calories 114, fat 9.2, fiber 3.6, carbs 6.3, protein 4.5

Paprika Chicken Bowl

Prep time: 10 minutes

Cooking time: 20 minutes

Servings: 2

Ingredients:

- 1 cup cremini mushrooms, sliced
- 10 oz chicken breast, skinless, boneless, chopped
- ½ cup heavy cream
- 1 teaspoon salt
- ½ teaspoon ground paprika
- ½ teaspoon cayenne pepper
- 1 tablespoon coconut oil

Directions:

1. Melt coconut oil in the instant pot on sauté mode.
2. Add cremini mushrooms and sauté them for 5 minutes.
3. After this, add chopped chicken breast.
4. Sprinkle the ingredients with salt, ground paprika, and cayenne pepper.
5. Cook them for 5 minutes more.
6. Then add heavy cream and close the lid.
7. Cook the meal on poultry mode for 10 minutes.

Nutrition value/serving: calories 336, fat 21.6, fiber 0.5, carbs 2.9, protein 31.7

Creamy Broccoli Soup

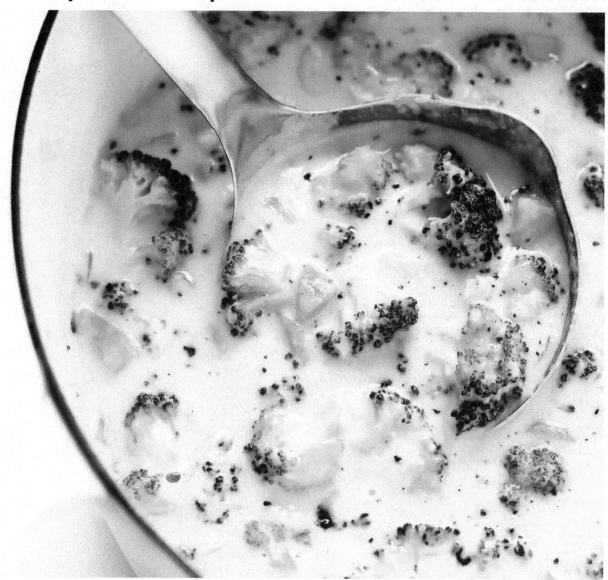

Prep time: 20 minutes

Cooking time: 5 minutes

Servings: 3

Ingredients:

- 1 cup chicken broth
- 1 cup heavy cream
- 1 teaspoon xanthan gum

- 2 cups broccoli, chopped
- ½ cup cheddar cheese, shredded
- ½ teaspoon salt
- 1 teaspoon ground black pepper
- ½ teaspoon chili flakes
- 1 teaspoon ground cumin

Directions:

1. Pour chicken broth and heavy cream in the instant pot.

2. Add broccoli, salt, ground black pepper, chili flakes, and ground cumin.

3. Close and seal the lid.

4. Cook the mixture on manual mode (high pressure) for 5 minutes.

5. Then allow the natural pressure release for 10 minutes and open the lid.

6. Add xanthan gum and blend the soup with the help of the immersion blender.

7. Ladle the soup in the bowls and top with cheddar cheese.

Nutrition value/serving: calories 252, fat 21.9, fiber 1.8, carbs 6.5, protein 9

Zucchini Pot Roast

Prep time: 10 minutes
Cooking time: 60 minutes
Servings: 4

Ingredients:

- 1-pound beef chuck pot roast, chopped
- 1 cup turnip, chopped
- 1 cup zucchini, chopped
- 1 garlic clove, diced
- 1 teaspoon salt
- 1 teaspoon coconut aminos
- 1 teaspoon ground black pepper
- 1 teaspoon butter
- 2 cups of water

Directions:

1. Put all ingredients in the instant pot and close the lid.
2. Set meat mode and cook the meal for 60 minutes.
3. When the time is over, open the lid and stir the ingredients carefully with the help of the spoon.

Nutrition value/serving: calories 269, fat 10.5, fiber 1.1, carbs 3.6, protein 38.2

Ham Mix with Green Beans

Prep time: 10 minutes
Cooking time: 6 minutes
Servings: 3

Ingredients:

- 2 cups green beans, chopped
- 7 oz ham, chopped
- ½ white onion, chopped
- 1 teaspoon olive oil
- ½ teaspoon salt
- ½ teaspoon ground nutmeg
- 1 cup water, for cooking

Directions:

1. Pour water and insert the steamer rack in the instant pot.

2. Place the green bean, ham, and onion in the rack and close the lid.

3. Cook the ingredients on steam mode for 6 minutes.

4. Then make a quick pressure release and transfer the ingredients in the big bowl.

5. Sprinkle them with ground nutmeg, salt, and olive oil. Stir well.

Nutrition value/serving: calories 153, fat 7.5, fiber 3.8, carbs 9.7, protein 12.5

Ginger Ham

Prep time: 10 minutes

Cooking time: 12 minutes

Servings: 5

Ingredients:

- 1-pound spiral ham, sliced
- 1 tablespoon Erythritol
- 2 tablespoons butter, melted
- ½ teaspoon minced ginger
- 1 teaspoon mustard
- 1 cup water, for cooking

Directions:

1.   In the shallow bowl combine together Erythritol, butter, minced ginger, and mustard.

2.   Then pour water and insert the trivet in the instant pot.

3.   Line the trivet with foil.

4.   Brush the spiral ham with butter mixture generously and transfer the ham in the instant pot.

5.   Cook the ham on manual mode (high pressure) for 12 minutes.

6.   When the time is over, make a quick pressure release and open the lid.

7.   Place the cooked spiral ham in the serving plate.

Nutrition value/serving: calories 237, fat 16.6, fiber 0.1, carbs 7.6, protein 17.3

Curry Soup

Prep time: 10 minutes

Cooking time: 13 minutes

Servings: 4

Ingredients:

- 2 cups of coconut milk
- 2 cups of water
- 1 teaspoon dried lemongrass
- 1 tablespoon lemon juice
- 1 teaspoon curry paste
- ½ cup white mushrooms, chopped
- 1 teaspoon butter

Directions:

1. Melt the butter in sauté mode.
2. Add mushrooms and sauté them for 3 minutes.
3. Then stir the vegetables and add lemongrass, lemon juice, and curry paste.
4. Add water and coconut milk. Stir the mixture until the curry paste is dissolved.
5. Close the lid and cook the soup on soup mode for 10 minutes.

Nutrition value/serving: calories 296, fat 30.4, fiber 2.8, carbs 7.5, protein 3.1

Ground Beef and Cabbage

Prep time: 10 minutes
Cooking time: 43 minutes
Servings: 2

Ingredients:
- 10 oz corned beef
- ½ teaspoon ground nutmeg
- ¼ teaspoon ground black pepper
- ¼ teaspoon ground paprika
- ¾ teaspoon salt
- 1 teaspoon dried cilantro
- 1 cup chicken broth
- 1 cup cabbage, chopped
- 1 teaspoon butter

Directions:
1. Rub the corned beef with ground nutmeg, ground black pepper, ground paprika, salt, and dried cilantro.
2. Place the meat in the instant pot. Add chicken broth and cook it on manual mode (high pressure) for 40 minutes.
3. When the time is over, make a quick pressure release and open the lid.
4. Shred the corned beef with the help of the fork and add chopped cabbage and butter.

5.   Cook the meal on manual (high pressure) for 3 minutes more.

6.   When the time is over, make a quick pressure release.

7.   Stir the cooked meal well.

Nutrition value/serving: calories 290, fat 20.6, fiber 1.2, carbs 3.1, protein 22

Lazy Chicken Mix

Prep time: 10 minutes
Cooking time: 45 minutes
Servings: 2

Ingredients:
- 3 oz chicken fillet, chopped
- 4 oz pork chops, chopped
- 4 oz beef sirloin, chopped
- 1 onion, chopped
- 1 teaspoon tomato paste
- 1 teaspoon dried rosemary
- 1 cup of water
- ½ teaspoon salt
- 1 teaspoon olive oil

Directions:
1. Preheat the olive oil on sauté mode.
2. Then add chicken, pork chops, and beef sirloin.
3. Add onion and cook the ingredients for 3 minutes.
4. Then stir them well and add tomato paste, dried rosemary, water, and salt.
5. Stir it well until tomato paste is dissolved.
6. Then close the lid and cook the meat mix on meat mode for 40 minutes.

Nutrition value/serving: calories 414, fat 23.3, fiber 1.6, carbs 6, protein 43

Creamy Chicken Salad

Prep time: 10 minutes
Cooking time: 12 minutes
Servings: 4

Ingredients:
- 9 oz Chinese cabbage, shredded
- 10 oz chicken fillet
- ½ teaspoon lemon juice
- ¼ cup heavy cream
- 1 teaspoon white pepper
- ½ cup of water
- ½ teaspoon salt
- ½ teaspoon ground turmeric
- ¼ teaspoon dried sage
- 1 tablespoon cream cheese
- 1 tablespoon sour cream
- ½ teaspoon dried dill

Directions:

1. Rub the chicken fillet with white pepper, salt, ground turmeric, and dried sage.

2. Place it in the instant pot.

3. Add water and heavy cream. Close and seal the lid. Cook the chicken on manual mode (high pressure) for 12 minutes. Then make a quick pressure release.

4. Remove the chicken fillet from the instant pot and shred it.

5. Put the shredded chicken in the salad bowl.

6. Add sour cream and cream cheese in the instant pot (to the cream mixture).

7. Then add dill and stir it.

8. Sprinkle the salad with lemon juice and ½ of the cream mixture from the instant pot. Mix up the salad well.

Nutrition value/serving: calories 187, fat 9.7, fiber 0.9, carbs 2.4, protein 22

Curry Soup

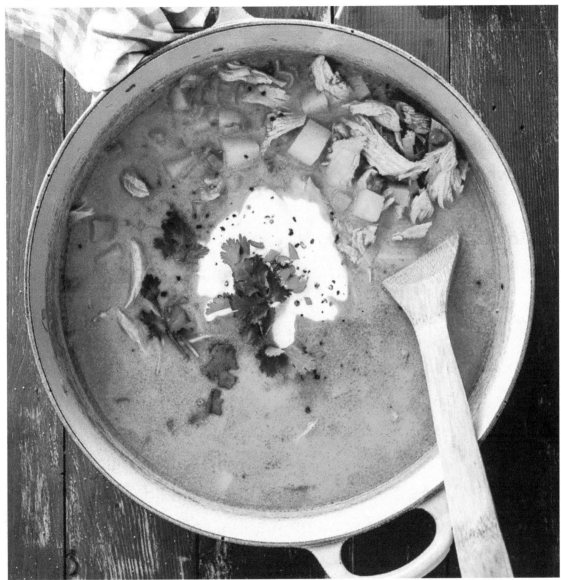

Prep time: 10 minutes

Cooking time: 30 minutes

Servings: 4

Ingredients:

- 1-pound beef sirloin, chopped
- 1 teaspoon curry powder
- 1 cup of coconut milk

- 3 cups of water
- 1 cup snap beans
- ½ teaspoon salt
- ½ teaspoon paprika
- 1 chili pepper, chopped
- 1 tablespoon coconut oil
- 1 white onion, diced

Directions:

1. Mix up together beef sirloin with curry powder, salt, and paprika.

2. Then put coconut oil in the instant pot and heat it up on sauté mode for 2 minutes.

3. Add beef sirloin and cook it on sauté mode for 10 minutes. Stir it from time to time.

4. After this, add water and coconut milk.

5. Add chili pepper and close the lid.

6. Cook the soup on manual mode (high pressure) for 15 minutes.

7. Then make a quick pressure release and open the lid.

8. Add snap beans and onion.

9. Cook the soup for 2 minutes more on manual mode (high pressure). Then make a quick pressure release.

Nutrition value/serving: calories 403, fat 25, fiber 3.2, carbs 8.9, protein 36.8

Conclusion

Being an excellent service both for immediate pot beginners and knowledgeable instant pot users this immediate pot cookbook boosts your day-to-day food preparation. It makes you look like a professional and cook like a pro. Thanks to the Immediate Pot component, this cookbook assists you with preparing straightforward and tasty meals for any budget. Satisfy everybody with hearty suppers, nutritious breakfasts, sweetest desserts, as well as enjoyable treats. Despite if you cook for one or prepare bigger sections-- there's a service for any type of feasible cooking circumstance. Boost your methods on how to cook in one of the most effective means making use of just your split second pot, this recipe book, and some perseverance to find out quick. Valuable ideas and also methods are discreetly incorporated into every recipe to make your household request new meals time and time again. Vegan options, solutions for meat-eaters and extremely satisfying ideas to unify the entire household at the same table. Consuming in your home is a common experience, as well as it can be so great to fulfill completely at the end of the day. Master your Instant Pot as well as take advantage of this brand-new experience beginning today!